STOMACH SURGERY RECOVERY

A Comprehensive Guide To Optimal Surgery Recovery Nutrition, Featuring Healing Recipes, Meal Plans, And Expert Tips For Long-Term Wellness

ALLAN FREDA

Contents

ABOUT THIS BOOK

This is a comprehensive guidebook dedicated to aiding individuals in their journey toward optimal recovery after undergoing stomach surgery.

This book delves into the essential aspects of post-surgery nutrition, emphasizing the significance of proper dietary choices in facilitating healing and promoting long-term wellness.

Inside this invaluable resource, readers will discover a wealth of information tailored to support their recovery journey. From healing recipes designed to provide essential nutrients and aid in the healing process to meticulously crafted meal plans, this book offers practical solutions for maintaining a balanced diet post-surgery.

Moreover, "Stomach Surgery Recovery" doesn't just stop at nutrition. It also provides expert tips and guidance from healthcare professionals to help individuals navigate the challenges of recovery effectively.

By incorporating evidence-based strategies and expert advice, this book equips readers with the knowledge and tools necessary to optimize their recovery journey and foster long-term wellness.

Whether you're preparing for stomach surgery or are currently in the recovery phase, this guide serves as a reliable companion, offering invaluable insights and resources to support your journey toward a healthier, happier life.

INTRODUCTION

Understanding Stomach Surgery Recovery:

Stomach surgery, whether it involves procedures like gastric bypass, gastrectomy, or other forms of abdominal surgery, is a significant medical intervention that requires careful consideration both before and after the operation. Recovery from stomach surgery can vary widely depending on the type of surgery performed, the individual's overall health, and any underlying conditions.

However, certain general principles and guidelines apply to most cases of stomach surgery recovery.

Post-surgery, patients often experience a range of physical and emotional challenges.

These may include pain, swelling, limited mobility, changes in appetite, digestive issues, and feelings of fatigue or weakness. Moreover, depending on the extent of the surgery and its purpose, patients may also need to adapt to significant changes in their dietary habits and nutritional intake. Proper nutrition plays a crucial role in the recovery process, as it helps support healing, replenish vital nutrients, maintain energy levels, and prevent complications.

In addition to physical recovery, it's essential to address the psychological and emotional aspects of recuperation. Patients may experience anxiety, depression, or frustration during the recovery period, especially if they encounter unexpected setbacks or challenges. Support from healthcare professionals, family members, and peers can be invaluable in navigating these emotional hurdles and maintaining a positive outlook on the recovery journey.

The recovery period following stomach surgery is a critical phase that requires careful attention to nutrition and dietary choices. This comprehensive cookbook aims to provide patients with the guidance, resources, and support they need to optimize their recovery journey through tailored nutrition strategies, healing recipes, meal plans, and expert tips.

By incorporating evidence-based nutritional principles and practical advice from healthcare professionals, nutritionists, and culinary experts, this cookbook offers a holistic approach to post-surgery recovery. Whether you're recovering from gastric bypass, gastrectomy, or other stomach surgeries, the recipes and meal plans included are designed to support healing, promote digestive health, and enhance overall well-being.

In addition to delicious and nutritious recipes, this cookbook features meal planning tips, grocery shopping guides, and food preparation techniques to help streamline the recovery process and make mealtime more manageable. From soothing soups and smoothies to protein-packed meals and nutrient-rich snacks, each recipe is carefully crafted to provide the essential nutrients and energy needed for optimal recovery.

Furthermore, this cookbook addresses common dietary challenges and concerns faced by patients during the recovery period, such as managing portion sizes, adjusting to new eating habits, and incorporating dietary restrictions or modifications. With practical advice and creative solutions, it empowers patients to make informed choices about their nutrition and navigate the post-surgery recovery journey with confidence.

Whether you're a patient recovering from stomach surgery, a caregiver supporting a loved one, or a healthcare professional seeking resources for your patients, this cookbook serves as a valuable tool for promoting healing, wellness, and long-term success. By prioritizing nutrition and embracing a nourishing approach to food, individuals can accelerate their recovery, minimize complications, and pave the way for a healthier future.

CHAPTER 1
PREPARING YOUR KITCHEN

Before delving into the realm of stomach surgery recovery nutrition, it's crucial to set the stage for success by preparing your kitchen adequately.

This initial step lays the foundation for a seamless transition into a nourishing post-surgery diet.

By ensuring that your kitchen is equipped with essential tools, stocked with appropriate pantry staples, and organized with effective meal-planning strategies, you can streamline the recovery process and optimize your nutritional intake for enhanced healing and long-term wellness.

Essential Kitchen Tools

Investing in the right kitchen tools can significantly simplify the preparation of nutrient-rich meals while minimizing physical strain during the recovery period. Key essentials include:

1.   **Blender or Food Processor**: A high-quality blender or food processor enables the easy creation of smoothies, soups, and purees, which are often recommended during the initial stages of stomach surgery recovery. These appliances facilitate the consumption of nutrient-dense foods in a form that is gentle on the digestive system.

2.   **Immersion Blender**: Particularly useful for blending soups directly in the pot, an immersion blender offers convenience and versatility in meal preparation, eliminating the need for transferring hot liquids to a separate blender.

3.   **Sharp Knives**: Sharp knives promote efficiency and safety in the kitchen, allowing for precise slicing and chopping of fruits, vegetables, and other ingredients. Maintaining sharpness reduces the risk of accidents and ensures a smoother cooking process.

4.   **Food Scale**: Precision in portion control is paramount during the recovery phase, making a food scale an invaluable tool for accurately

measuring ingredients and monitoring serving sizes as recommended by healthcare professionals.

5. **Steamer Basket**: Steaming is a gentle cooking method that helps retain the nutritional integrity of foods while preserving their natural flavors and textures. A steamer basket facilitates the preparation of tender vegetables, fish, and lean proteins without the need for added fats or oils.

6. **Slow Cooker or Instant Pot**: These versatile appliances are ideal for preparing wholesome meals with minimal effort, allowing busy individuals to enjoy nutritious, home-cooked dishes without extensive hands-on cooking time.

7. **Measuring Cups and Spoons**: Consistent measurement of ingredients is essential for following recipes and adhering to dietary guidelines post-surgery. Measuring cups and spoons ensure accuracy and consistency in portion sizes, aiding in effective nutrient management.

By equipping your kitchen with these essential tools, you can streamline the cooking process and enhance the accessibility of nourishing meals throughout your stomach surgery recovery journey.

Stocking Your Pantry

A well-stocked pantry is the cornerstone of a nutritious and varied diet, especially during periods of recovery when physical mobility may be limited. Prioritize the inclusion of nutrient-dense foods that align with your post-surgery dietary recommendations, focusing on items that are easy to prepare and gentle on the digestive system. Essential pantry staples for stomach surgery recovery include:

1.   **Whole Grains**: Opt for easily digestible whole grains such as quinoa, brown rice, oats, and whole grain pasta, which provide essential nutrients such as fiber, vitamins, and minerals to support healing and digestion.

2.   **Protein Sources**: Incorporate lean protein sources such as canned beans, lentils, tofu, tempeh, canned tuna or salmon, and nut butter to

promote tissue repair, muscle recovery, and overall strength during the recovery process.

3.   **Healthy Fats**: Choose heart-healthy fats such as olive oil, avocado oil, nuts, seeds, and avocado to support inflammation reduction, nutrient absorption, and overall cardiovascular health post-surgery.

4.   **Low-FODMAP Options**: If advised by your healthcare provider, consider stocking low-FODMAP foods such as lactose-free dairy products, gluten-free grains, and non-cruciferous vegetables to minimize gastrointestinal discomfort and promote digestive tolerance.

5.   **Fruits and Vegetables**: Opt for soft, ripe fruits and cooked or steamed vegetables that are rich in vitamins, minerals, and antioxidants. Applesauce, mashed bananas, steamed carrots, and spinach are excellent choices for gentle digestion and optimal nutrient absorption.

6.   **Hydration**: Stay hydrated by keeping a variety of fluids on hand, including water, herbal

teas, low-sodium broth, and electrolyte-rich beverages. Adequate hydration is essential for supporting healing, preventing dehydration, and maintaining overall health.

7. **Herbs and Spices**: Enhance the flavor of your meals with an assortment of herbs, spices, and seasonings such as ginger, turmeric, cinnamon, basil, and mint, which not only add depth to dishes but also offer potential anti-inflammatory and digestive benefits.

Regularly assess and replenish your pantry supplies to ensure that you have a diverse selection of nutritious ingredients readily available for meal preparation and snacking during your stomach surgery recovery.

Meal Planning Tips

Effective meal planning is essential for optimizing nutrition, managing dietary restrictions, and promoting consistency in eating habits throughout the recovery process. Consider the following tips to streamline meal planning and preparation:

1.   **Create a Weekly Meal Schedule**: Plan your meals for the week ahead, taking into account any dietary guidelines provided by your healthcare team. Structure your meals to include a balance of protein, carbohydrates, healthy fats, and vegetables to support optimal healing and nutrition.

2.   **Batch Cooking**: Prepare large batches of staple foods such as grains, proteins, and vegetables at the beginning of the week to streamline meal assembly and minimize daily cooking time. Store cooked ingredients in portioned containers for easy access and quick meal assembly.

3.   **Include Variety**: Incorporate a variety of flavors, textures, and colors into your meals to keep them interesting and enjoyable. Experiment with different ingredients, cuisines, and cooking methods to prevent culinary monotony and enhance nutritional diversity.

4.   **Listen to Your Body**: Pay attention to your body's hunger cues, energy levels, and digestive responses when planning meals and portion sizes. Eat mindfully and intuitively, stopping when you feel satisfied and avoiding overeating or undereating.

5.   **Plan for Snacks**: Keep a selection of nutrient-dense snacks on hand to satisfy hunger between meals and prevent excessive grazing or reliance on less nutritious options. Opt for portable snacks such as Greek yogurt, fresh fruit, nuts, and whole grain crackers for convenient, on-the-go nourishment.

6.   **Consult with a Registered Dietitian**: If you have specific dietary concerns or restrictions related to your surgery or medical condition, seek guidance from a registered dietitian or nutritionist who can provide personalized recommendations and support for your recovery journey.

By implementing these meals planning strategies and incorporating nutritious pantry staples into your daily routine, you can support optimal healing, nourishment, and long-term wellness following stomach surgery.

Take proactive steps to prepare your kitchen, stock your pantry, and plan your meals with intention, prioritizing nutrient-rich foods and mindful eating practices to facilitate a smooth and successful recovery process.

CHAPTER 2
NUTRITIONAL GUIDELINES

Understanding Nutritional Needs Post-Surgery

Post-surgery nutrition plays a crucial role in the recovery process, as it aids in wound healing, reduces the risk of infection, and supports overall health. Understanding the nutritional needs during this period is paramount for a successful recovery. Following surgery, the body requires an increased intake of certain nutrients to promote tissue repair, boost the immune system, and restore energy levels. Additionally, factors such as the type of surgery, individual health status, and any pre-existing conditions must be considered when planning a post-surgery diet.

Macronutrients and Micronutrients

Macronutrients, including carbohydrates, proteins, and fats, are essential for providing energy and supporting various bodily functions.

In the context of surgery recovery, each macronutrient plays a distinct role.

Carbohydrates serve as the body's primary source of energy, aiding in cellular repair and preventing muscle loss. However, it's essential to focus on complex carbohydrates, such as whole grains and fruits, to maintain stable blood sugar levels and avoid energy crashes. Proteins are crucial for tissue repair and immune function, making them vital components of a post-surgery diet.

Lean sources of protein, such as poultry, fish, beans, and legumes, should be incorporated into meals to support healing and prevent muscle wasting.

Micronutrients, including vitamins and minerals, are equally important for surgery recovery, as they play key roles in various physiological processes. Vitamin C, for example, is essential for collagen synthesis, which is critical for wound healing.

Foods rich in vitamin C, such as citrus fruits, strawberries, and bell peppers, should be included in the diet to support tissue repair and reduce the risk of infection.

Similarly, adequate intake of zinc, found in foods like meat, seafood, nuts, and seeds, is essential for immune function and wound healing. Other micronutrients, such as vitamin A, vitamin D, and iron, also play important roles in the recovery process and should be prioritized in the post-surgery diet.

Portion Control Tips

While ensuring adequate nutrient intake is important for surgery recovery, portion control is equally crucial to prevent overeating and promote optimal healing. After surgery, appetite may fluctuate, and digestion may be impaired, making it necessary to pay attention to portion sizes.

Instead of large meals, opt for smaller, more frequent meals throughout the day to provide a steady supply of nutrients without overwhelming the digestive system. Additionally, focus on nutrient-dense foods that pack a powerful nutritional punch without excess calories. Incorporating plenty of fruits, vegetables, lean proteins, and whole grains into meals can help ensure adequate nutrient intake while controlling portion sizes.

Furthermore, mindful eating practices, such as chewing slowly and Savoring each bite, can aid digestion and promote satiety, preventing the urge to overeat. Avoiding distractions during meals, such as watching TV or scrolling through devices, can also help foster mindful eating habits and prevent mindless overeating. Additionally, listening to hunger and fullness cues and stopping eating when satisfied can prevent discomfort and promote optimal digestion. By implementing portion control tips and mindful eating practices, individuals can support their recovery journey and optimize their nutritional intake for accelerated healing and long-term wellness.

CHAPTER 3
<u>HEALING RECIPES</u>

Recovery from stomach surgery is a crucial process that requires careful attention to nutrition to facilitate healing and prevent complications.

The journey to optimal recovery involves consuming nutrient-dense foods that are easily digestible, soothing to the stomach, and promote tissue repair. In this comprehensive guide to optimal surgery recovery nutrition, we delve into various healing recipes designed to support your recovery journey. From liquid and pureed recipes to texture-modified dishes, protein-packed meals, and energy-boosting snacks, each category serves a specific purpose in aiding recovery and promoting overall well-being.

Liquid and Pureed Recipes

Following stomach surgery, especially in the immediate post-operative phase, consuming liquid and pureed foods is often recommended to allow the digestive system to rest and gradually reintroduce nutrients. Liquid and pureed recipes are gentle on the stomach, easy to swallow, and provide essential nutrients necessary for healing. These recipes typically include soups, broths, smoothies, and pureed fruits and vegetables. Incorporating protein sources such as Greek yogurt, tofu, or protein powder into smoothies can help maintain muscle mass and support tissue repair. Additionally, adding healthy fats like avocado or nut butter can provide essential calories for energy.

Soft Foods Recipes

As recovery progresses and the digestive system begins to tolerate more substantial foods, soft foods become an integral part of the diet. Soft food recipes include dishes that are soft, easy to chew, and gentle on the stomach. Examples of soft foods include mashed potatoes, steamed vegetables, scrambled eggs, cooked grains like rice or quinoa, and tender cooked meats or fish.

These foods provide a wider variety of nutrients while still being gentle enough for a healing stomach. It's essential to focus on incorporating lean proteins, complex carbohydrates, and healthy fats into soft food recipes to support the body's recovery process effectively.

Texture-Modified Dishes

For individuals who may have difficulty swallowing or have specific dietary restrictions following stomach surgery, texture-modified dishes can provide alternative options while still meeting nutritional needs. Texture-modified recipes often involve altering the consistency or texture of foods to make them easier to swallow or digest. This can include pureeing, chopping, or blending foods to create smoother textures or avoiding foods that are hard or crunchy. Examples of texture-modified dishes include blended soups, mashed vegetables, pureed fruits, and finely minced meats.

These recipes ensure that individuals with specific dietary challenges can still enjoy a variety of nutritious foods while promoting healing and recovery.

Protein-Packed Meals

Protein is an essential nutrient for post-surgery recovery as it plays a vital role in tissue repair, immune function, and muscle maintenance. Protein-packed meals focus on incorporating high-quality protein sources into the diet to support healing and prevent muscle loss. Examples of protein-packed meals include grilled chicken or fish with steamed vegetables, tofu stir-fry with quinoa, lentil soup with whole-grain bread, or Greek yogurt with berries and nuts. It's important to include a variety of protein sources such as lean meats, poultry, fish, legumes, dairy, and plant-based proteins to ensure adequate intake of essential amino acids and promote optimal recovery.

Energy-Boosting Snacks

During the recovery process, maintaining energy levels is essential for supporting healing and preventing fatigue.

 Energy-boosting snacks provide a quick and convenient way to replenish energy stores and satisfy hunger between meals.

These snacks are typically nutrient-dense, containing a balance of carbohydrates, protein, and healthy fats to provide sustained energy.

Examples of energy-boosting snacks include a trail mix with nuts and dried fruits, Greek yogurt with honey and granola, whole-grain crackers with cheese, hummus with carrot sticks, or a banana with almond butter. Incorporating these snacks into your recovery diet can help maintain energy levels throughout the day and support overall well-being.

incorporating healing recipes into your post-stomach surgery recovery plan is essential for promoting optimal healing, preventing complications, and supporting long-term wellness.

Whether you're enjoying liquid and pureed recipes in the early stages of recovery or transitioning to soft foods, texture-modified dishes, protein-packed meals, and energy-boosting snacks as you progress, focusing on nutrient-dense foods is key. Consult with a healthcare professional or registered dietitian to tailor your nutrition plan to your individual needs and ensure a smooth and successful recovery journey.

CHAPTER 4
FLAVORFUL SOUPS AND BROTHS

Flavorful soups and broths play a pivotal role in the recovery process following stomach surgery, providing vital nutrients, hydration, and comfort during the healing journey. Among the myriad options, nourishing bone broths, comforting vegetable soups, and creamy pureed soups stand out as particularly beneficial for patients recuperating from surgical procedures on the stomach. Understanding the importance of these components in post-operative recovery, as well as their nutritional value and ease of digestion can significantly contribute to optimal healing outcomes.

Nourishing Bone Broths:
Nourishing bone broths are renowned for their healing properties, making them a staple in post-surgery recovery diets.

Rich in essential nutrients such as collagen, gelatin, amino acids, and minerals like calcium and magnesium, bone broths offer a plethora of benefits for individuals recovering from stomach surgery. Collagen and gelatin, derived from simmering bones and connective tissues, aid in tissue repair and regeneration, crucial for healing surgical incisions and promoting overall gastrointestinal health.

Amino acids such as glycine and proline support immune function, reduce inflammation, and facilitate the absorption of nutrients, essential for the body's recovery process. Additionally, the presence of minerals helps replenish electrolytes and supports bone density, addressing potential deficiencies that may arise during the recovery period. Incorporating nourishing bone broths into the post-operative diet not only provides essential nutrients but also offers comforting warmth and hydration, aiding in the restoration of energy levels and overall well-being.

Comforting vegetable soups are a delightful addition to the post-surgery recovery diet, offering a myriad of vitamins, minerals, and antioxidants essential for healing and overall health.

Packed with nutrient-dense vegetables such as carrots, celery, spinach, and kale, these soups provide a wide array of essential nutrients that support immune function, promote tissue repair and aid in digestion.

The abundance of vitamins A, C, and K found in vegetables contributes to the body's healing process by supporting collagen production, boosting immunity, and enhancing wound healing. Additionally, the fiber content in vegetable aids in digestion, regulates bowel movements, and promotes gut health, crucial for individuals recovering from stomach surgery.

By incorporating comforting vegetable soups into the diet, patients can enjoy a delicious and nourishing way to replenish vital nutrients, support healing, and promote overall well-being during the recovery period.

Creamy Pureed Soups:

Creamy pureed soups offer a smooth and easily digestible option for individuals recovering from stomach surgery, providing essential nutrients without putting strain on the digestive system. Made by blending cooked vegetables, broth, and other wholesome ingredients to a smooth consistency, these soups are gentle on the stomach, making them ideal for individuals with limited appetite or sensitive digestive systems post-surgery.

The creamy texture of pureed soups adds a comforting element to the diet, providing a source of nourishment and hydration during the recovery process. By incorporating nutrient-rich ingredients such as sweet potatoes, squash, lentils, or beans, creamy pureed soups offer a balanced combination of carbohydrates, protein, and fats, essential for supporting energy levels, muscle repair, and overall recovery.

Additionally, the versatility of pureed soups allows for creative flavor combinations and nutrient-rich additions, ensuring a satisfying and nourishing meal option for individuals on the path to healing.

In summary, flavorful soups and broths, including nourishing bone broths, comforting vegetable soups, and creamy pureed soups, are invaluable components of the post-surgery recovery diet. These nutrient-dense options provide essential vitamins, minerals, and antioxidants necessary for tissue repair, immune function, and overall well-being. By incorporating these healing recipes into the recovery plan, patients can accelerate the healing process, replenish vital nutrients, and promote long-term wellness following stomach surgery.

CHAPTER 5
GENTLE AND DIGESTIBLE MEALS

In the critical phase of post-stomach surgery recovery, the choice of meals plays a pivotal role in facilitating healing and restoring nutritional balance. The digestive system undergoes significant stress during and after surgery, necessitating a shift towards gentle and easily digestible meals.

This transition is essential to minimize discomfort, promote optimal nutrient absorption, and support the body's healing processes.

Bland but Tasty Dishes

Following stomach surgery, particularly procedures like gastrectomy or gastric bypass, patients often experience changes in their digestive capabilities and tolerance to certain foods. Therefore, opting for bland but tasty dishes becomes imperative.

These dishes should offer subtle flavors without overwhelming the sensitive gastrointestinal tract. Boiled or steamed lean meats such as chicken or fish can serve as excellent protein sources. Pairing them with simple carbohydrates like rice or potatoes can provide energy without causing digestive distress.

Additionally, incorporating mild herbs and spices like ginger, parsley, or basil can enhance flavor without irritating the stomach lining. Utilizing low-fat cooking methods such as baking, broiling, or poaching further ensures that the meals remain gentle on the stomach while still being palatable.

Easy-to-Digest Entrees

Choosing easy-to-digest entrees is essential for promoting comfort and aiding the recovery process after stomach surgery. Opting for tender and lean protein sources such as tofu, eggs, or well-cooked legumes can provide essential amino acids without burdening the digestive system. These proteins are easier to break down compared to their higher-fat or tougher counterparts, reducing the risk of post-meal discomfort or complications.

Moreover, incorporating soft, cooked vegetables like carrots, zucchini, or spinach can offer vital vitamins, minerals, and fiber without causing undue stress on the digestive tract. Steaming or sautéing these vegetables until they reach a tender consistency can further enhance digestibility while preserving their nutritional value. Pairing these easy-to-digest entrees with small portions of complex carbohydrates like quinoa or whole-grain bread can provide sustained energy levels without overwhelming the stomach.

Delicate Vegetable Sides

Incorporating delicate vegetable sides into post-stomach surgery meals is crucial for ensuring a well-rounded and nutritionally balanced diet.

These sides should focus on providing essential nutrients and fiber while being gentle on the digestive system. Opting for cooked rather than raw vegetables can help mitigate digestive discomfort, as cooking breaks down tough fibers and makes them easier to digest. Vegetables such as squash, bell peppers, and green beans can be steamed or roasted until they reach a soft and tender consistency, making them suitable choices for individuals recovering from stomach surgery.

Additionally, incorporating root vegetables like sweet potatoes or beets can provide valuable vitamins, minerals, and antioxidants, supporting overall health and immune function during the recovery process. Pairing these delicate vegetable sides with lean proteins and whole grains can create well-balanced meals that promote healing and long-term wellness.

In summary, prioritizing gentle and digestible meals is essential for facilitating optimal recovery after stomach surgery. By focusing on bland but tasty dishes, easy-to-digest entrees, and delicate vegetable sides, individuals can support their healing journey while enjoying nourishing and satisfying meals.

Incorporating these strategies into post-surgery nutrition plans can accelerate healing, minimize discomfort, and promote long-term wellness and quality of life.

CHAPTER 6

SMOOTHIES AND SHAKES

Smoothies and shakes play a pivotal role in the recovery process after stomach surgery. They offer a convenient and efficient way to deliver essential nutrients to the body, particularly when solid foods may be difficult to consume. This comprehensive guide aims to explore the importance of smoothies and shakes in post-surgery recovery, emphasizing protein-packed smoothies, nutrient-rich shakes, and fiber-filled blends.

Protein-Packed Smoothies: Protein is a crucial component of the healing process following stomach surgery. It aids in tissue repair, muscle rebuilding, and overall recovery. Protein-packed smoothies provide a convenient and easily digestible source of this essential nutrient. Incorporating high-quality protein sources such as Greek yogurt, whey protein powder, tofu, or nut butter into smoothies can help promote healing and prevent muscle loss during the recovery period. Additionally, adding fruits like berries, bananas, or mangoes not only enhances the flavor but also provides vitamins, minerals, and antioxidants necessary for optimal recovery.

Nutrient-Rich Shakes: Stomach surgery can often lead to nutrient deficiencies due to decreased food intake or impaired absorption.

Nutrient-rich shakes are a valuable tool in replenishing essential vitamins and minerals, promoting overall health and well-being.

These shakes can be fortified with ingredients such as leafy greens, avocado, chia seeds, or spirulina to boost their nutrient content.

Furthermore, incorporating liquid supplements or meal replacement powders specifically formulated for post-surgery recovery can ensure adequate nutrient intake without placing undue stress on the digestive system.

Fiber-Filled Blends: Maintaining regular bowel movements is essential for preventing complications such as constipation or bowel obstruction post-stomach surgery.

Fiber-filled blends can help support digestive health and alleviate gastrointestinal discomfort during the recovery process. Ingredients such as spinach, kale, flaxseeds, or psyllium husk can be added to smoothies and shakes to increase their fiber content. Additionally, incorporating fruits with edible skins like apples or pears can provide insoluble fiber, promoting bowel regularity and preventing constipation.

However, it's crucial to gradually increase fiber intake and stay hydrated to prevent any adverse effects on digestion.

In summary, incorporating smoothies and shakes into the post-stomach surgery recovery plan can significantly aid in the healing process and promote long-term wellness. Protein-packed smoothies, nutrient-rich shakes, and fiber-filled blends offer a convenient and effective way to deliver essential nutrients while supporting digestive health.

By experimenting with different ingredients and recipes, individuals can tailor their smoothies and shakes to meet their specific nutritional needs and preferences, facilitating a smooth and successful recovery journey.

CHAPTER 7
CUSTOMIZING YOUR DIET

In the journey towards recovery from stomach surgery, nutrition plays a pivotal role. A tailored diet plan can aid in optimal healing, alleviate discomfort, and promote long-term wellness. Customizing your diet post-stomach surgery involves understanding dietary restrictions and modifications, exploring vegan and vegetarian options, as well as incorporating gluten-free and dairy-free alternatives. By carefully selecting foods that are gentle on the stomach yet rich in essential nutrients, individuals can enhance their recovery process and foster overall well-being.

Dietary Restrictions and Modifications:

Following stomach surgery, individuals may encounter various dietary restrictions and modifications to accommodate the healing process and prevent complications.

One of the primary concerns is the need for easily digestible foods that minimize strain on the gastrointestinal system.

This often entails avoiding hard-to-digest foods such as fatty meats, spicy dishes, and foods high in fiber. Instead, focus is placed on incorporating soft, bland foods that are gentle on the stomach, such as cooked vegetables, lean proteins, and easily digestible grains.

Moreover, portion control becomes crucial as the stomach's capacity may be reduced post-surgery. Smaller, more frequent meals spread throughout the day can help prevent discomfort and promote better digestion. Additionally, it's essential to stay adequately hydrated by consuming fluids regularly, although it's advisable to avoid beverages that are carbonated or caffeinated, as they can potentially irritate the stomach lining.

Individuals recovering from stomach surgery may also need to adjust their diet to manage specific conditions that may have necessitated the surgery, such as gastroesophageal reflux disease (GERD) or ulcers. This may involve limiting acidic foods, caffeine, and spicy ingredients, which can exacerbate symptoms. Consulting with a healthcare provider or a registered dietitian can provide valuable guidance in tailoring the diet to individual needs and ensuring proper nutrition during the recovery period.

Vegan and Vegetarian Options:

For individuals adhering to a vegan or vegetarian lifestyle, maintaining adequate nutrition during the recovery phase of stomach surgery may require some adjustments. While plant-based diets offer numerous health benefits, they may also present challenges in meeting certain nutrient requirements, particularly protein, iron, calcium, and vitamin B12. However, with careful planning and consideration, vegan and vegetarian options can be incorporated into a post-surgery diet to promote healing and overall wellness.

Plant-based protein sources such as tofu, tempeh, legumes, nuts, and seeds can serve as excellent alternatives to meat and dairy products. Incorporating a variety of these protein-rich foods into meals can help meet daily protein needs and support tissue repair and recovery. Additionally, focusing on nutrient-dense whole foods such as fruits, vegetables, whole grains, and healthy fats can provide essential vitamins, minerals, and antioxidants necessary for optimal healing.

Furthermore, individuals following a vegan or vegetarian diet should pay particular attention to vitamin B12 intake, as this nutrient is primarily found in animal products. Fortified foods such as plant-based milk, nutritional yeast, and fortified cereals can help bridge this gap, or supplements may be necessary to ensure adequate levels of vitamin B12. Additionally, consuming foods rich in iron and vitamin C can enhance iron absorption and prevent deficiency, which is common in plant-based diets.

Gluten-Free and Dairy-Free Alternatives:

For individuals with gluten intolerance or sensitivity, as well as those with lactose intolerance or dairy allergies, navigating the post-surgery recovery period requires careful consideration of gluten-free and dairy-free alternatives. The protein gluten, which is present in wheat, barley, and rye, can cause negative reactions.

in individuals with celiac disease or gluten sensitivity, leading to inflammation and digestive discomfort. Similarly, lactose, a sugar found in dairy products, can cause digestive issues in individuals with lactose intolerance or dairy allergies.

Fortunately, there is a wide array of gluten-free and dairy-free alternatives available to accommodate these dietary restrictions. For individuals avoiding gluten, options such as gluten-free grains (e.g., rice, quinoa, millet), gluten-free bread, pasta, and flour blends can serve as substitutes for their gluten-containing counterparts. Additionally, naturally gluten-free foods such as fruits, vegetables, lean proteins, and legumes are safe and nutritious choices for a post-surgery diet.

Similarly, individuals avoiding dairy can opt for dairy-free alternatives such as plant-based milk (e.g., almond milk, soy milk, coconut milk), dairy-free yogurt, cheese, and ice cream made from nuts, seeds, or coconut. These alternatives provide essential nutrients such as calcium, vitamin D, and protein without the lactose or dairy proteins that can cause digestive issues. Furthermore, incorporating calcium-rich foods such as leafy greens, fortified non-dairy products, and calcium-fortified orange juice can help maintain bone health and support recovery.

 customizing your diet post-stomach surgery involves adapting to dietary restrictions and modifications, exploring vegan and vegetarian options, and incorporating gluten-free and dairy-free alternatives. By selecting foods that are gentle on the stomach, rich in essential nutrients, and tailored to individual needs, individuals can optimize their recovery process, alleviate discomfort, and promote long-term wellness. Consulting with healthcare professionals or registered dietitians can provide personalized guidance and support throughout the recovery journey, ensuring a smooth transition to a nourishing and sustainable diet for optimal healing and well-being.

CHAPTER 8

MANAGING SYMPTOMS

Managing symptoms such as nausea, preventing dumping syndrome, and alleviating digestive discomfort are crucial aspects of stomach surgery recovery. Patients undergoing stomach surgery, whether it's for weight loss purposes or to treat medical conditions like gastric ulcers or cancer, often face various challenges during the recovery period. These challenges can include nausea, dumping syndrome, and digestive discomfort, all of which can significantly impact the patient's quality of life and hinder their recovery progress. Therefore, it's essential to effectively manage these symptoms to promote optimal healing and ensure long-term wellness.

Dealing with Nausea:

Nausea is a common symptom experienced by many patients following stomach surgery. It can be caused by factors such as anesthesia, postoperative pain medications, changes in diet, and alterations in gastrointestinal function. Managing nausea effectively is crucial for ensuring patient comfort and facilitating the recovery process. One approach to dealing with nausea is to identify and avoid triggers that exacerbate the symptoms.

This may involve adjusting medication dosages, modifying the diet to include bland and easily digestible foods, and practicing relaxation techniques to alleviate stress and anxiety, which can worsen nausea. Additionally, staying hydrated is essential for preventing dehydration, which can worsen nausea. Sipping on clear fluids such as water, ginger tea, or electrolyte solutions can help soothe the stomach and alleviate symptoms. In some cases, anti-nausea medications may be prescribed by healthcare providers to provide relief for severe or persistent nausea.

Dumping syndrome is a common complication of stomach surgery, particularly procedures such as gastric bypass surgery.

It occurs when food moves too quickly from the stomach into the small intestine, leading to symptoms such as nausea, vomiting, diarrhea, dizziness, and weakness. Preventing dumping syndrome requires careful management of dietary intake and eating habits. Patients are advised to consume small, frequent meals throughout the day rather than large meals, which can overwhelm the digestive system and trigger symptoms.

Foods high in simple sugars, such as sweets, sugary beverages, and refined carbohydrates, should be avoided as they can exacerbate dumping syndrome. Instead, focusing on a balanced diet rich in lean proteins, complex carbohydrates, fiber, and healthy fats can help stabilize blood sugar levels and slow down gastric emptying, reducing the risk of dumping syndrome.

Eating meals slowly and chewing food thoroughly can also aid digestion and prevent symptoms.

Patients need to work closely with dietitians and healthcare providers to develop personalized meal plans that meet their nutritional needs while minimizing the risk of dumping syndrome.

Alleviating Digestive Discomfort:

Digestive discomfort is another common issue faced by patients during stomach surgery recovery. This can include symptoms such as bloating, gas, indigestion, and constipation, which can be caused by factors such as changes in diet, alterations in gastrointestinal anatomy, and side effects of medications. Alleviating digestive discomfort requires a multifaceted approach that addresses the underlying causes of symptoms.

Dietary modifications play a key role in managing digestive discomfort, with an emphasis on consuming foods that are easy to digest and gentle on the stomach. This may include incorporating probiotic-rich foods such as yogurt, kefir, and fermented vegetables to promote gut health and improve digestion. Increasing fiber intake through fruits, vegetables, whole grains, and legumes can help prevent constipation and regulate bowel movements. Additionally, staying hydrated by drinking plenty of water and herbal teas can promote regularity and ease digestive symptoms. In some cases, over-the-counter medications such as antacids, laxatives, or digestive enzymes may be recommended to provide relief for specific symptoms. However, patients need to consult with their healthcare providers before taking any medications, as they may interact with other medications or exacerbate underlying conditions. Overall, managing digestive discomfort requires a holistic approach that addresses diet, hydration, lifestyle factors, and, if necessary, medications to promote optimal gastrointestinal health and enhance the recovery process.

managing symptoms such as nausea, preventing dumping syndrome, and alleviating digestive discomfort are critical components of stomach surgery recovery. By identifying and addressing triggers, making dietary modifications, and implementing lifestyle changes, patients can effectively manage these symptoms and promote optimal healing and long-term wellness.

Working closely with healthcare providers, including surgeons, dietitians, and other members of the healthcare team, is essential for developing personalized strategies tailored to individual needs and optimizing the recovery process. With proper symptom management and support, patients can navigate the challenges of stomach surgery recovery with confidence and achieve positive outcomes for their health and well-being.

CHAPTER 9
REINTRODUCING SOLID FOODS

Reintroducing solid foods after stomach surgery is a crucial phase in the recovery process, requiring careful attention to ensure optimal healing and minimize complications. The transition from liquid or soft foods back to solids must be gradual and tailored to individual tolerance levels, taking into account the type of surgery performed and any dietary restrictions imposed by the healthcare provider. In this section, we will delve into the essential concepts surrounding the reintroduction of solid foods, offering practical tips for a smooth transition, methods for testing tolerance levels, and guidance on building a balanced plate to support healing and long-term wellness.

Gradual Transition Tips:

One of the primary considerations when reintroducing solid foods post-stomach surgery is the gradual transition from easily digestible liquids or soft foods to more complex solid foods.

This gradual approach helps the digestive system adapt to processing solid foods again, reducing the risk of discomfort, nausea, or digestive issues. Patients are typically advised to start with small portions of easily digestible foods, such as cooked vegetables, lean proteins, and whole grains, before gradually increasing the variety and complexity of foods in their diet.

It's essential to listen to your body during this transition phase and pay attention to any signs of discomfort or intolerance. Slowly increasing the texture and volume of solid foods allows the stomach to adjust gradually, minimizing the risk of complications such as dumping syndrome or postprandial discomfort. Patients should follow the guidance of their healthcare provider or dietitian regarding the pace and progression of the transition, as individual tolerance levels may vary based on factors such as the type of surgery performed and the extent of gastric resection.

Testing Tolerance Levels:

Testing tolerance levels is a critical aspect of reintroducing solid foods after stomach surgery, as it helps identify foods that may cause discomfort or trigger digestive issues. Patients are encouraged to keep a food diary to track their dietary intake and any associated symptoms, such as bloating, nausea, or diarrhea. By systematically reintroducing different food groups and observing their effects on digestion, patients can identify well-tolerated foods and those that may need to be avoided or consumed in moderation.

Certain foods may pose challenges for individuals recovering from stomach surgery, such as high-fat or high-fiber foods, spicy foods, or foods with tough textures. Patients should be cautious when reintroducing these foods and pay attention to how their body responds. Additionally, chewing food thoroughly and eating slowly can help facilitate digestion and reduce the risk of discomfort or digestive issues.

Building a Balanced Plate:

Building a balanced plate is essential for supporting healing and long-term wellness after stomach surgery. A balanced diet provides the essential nutrients needed for tissue repair, immune function, and overall health, while also promoting satiety and stable blood sugar levels.

When planning meals, patients should aim to include a variety of nutrient-dense foods from all food groups, including lean proteins, whole grains, fruits, vegetables, and healthy fats.

Protein is particularly important for healing and recovery after surgery, as it provides the building blocks for tissue repair and helps maintain muscle mass.

Patients should include a source of lean protein with each meal, such as poultry, fish, tofu, beans, or low-fat dairy products.

Whole grains, such as brown rice, quinoa, oats, and whole wheat bread, provide fiber and essential nutrients, while fruits and vegetables offer vitamins, minerals, and antioxidants to support immune function and overall health.

In addition to macronutrients, patients should pay attention to hydration and aim to drink plenty of fluids throughout the day, focusing on water and other low-calorie beverages. Adequate hydration is essential for digestion, nutrient absorption, and overall well-being. Patients should limit or avoid sugary beverages, carbonated drinks, and alcohol, as these can exacerbate digestive issues and hinder recovery.

reintroducing solid foods after stomach surgery requires a gradual transition, careful monitoring of tolerance levels, and a focus on building a balanced plate to support healing and long-term wellness.

By following these guidelines and working closely with healthcare providers and dietitians, patients can optimize their recovery and improve their overall quality of life post-surgery.

CHAPTER 10
LIFESTYLE TIPS FOR RECOVERY

Stomach surgery, whether it's for weight loss, treating a medical condition, or other reasons, demands careful attention not only during the procedure but also throughout the recovery phase. Lifestyle adjustments play a crucial role in ensuring a smooth recuperation process, aiding in optimal healing, and promoting long-term wellness.

 Here, we delve into essential lifestyle tips that encompass gentle exercise suggestions, stress management techniques, and rest and recovery practices.

Gentle Exercise Suggestions:
Engaging in appropriate physical activity post-stomach surgery is pivotal for enhancing circulation, preventing complications like blood clots, and maintaining muscle tone. However, it's

imperative to start with gentle exercises that don't strain the body excessively.

Walking stands out as one of the most accessible and beneficial exercises post-stomach surgery. Begin with short, leisurely walks, gradually increasing duration and intensity as tolerated. Swimming can also be an excellent low-impact option, providing a full-body workout without placing undue stress on the abdomen. Incorporating light stretching exercises can aid in maintaining flexibility and preventing stiffness, particularly crucial if mobility is restricted following surgery. Additionally, consult with a healthcare provider or physical therapist for personalized exercise recommendations tailored to your specific surgery and recovery progress.

Stress Management Techniques:

Managing stress is paramount for promoting healing and overall well-being during the recovery phase post-stomach surgery. Surgery itself can induce anxiety and stress, and coping with discomfort during recovery exacerbates these feelings. Employing effective stress management techniques can significantly alleviate these burdens. Mindfulness practices, such as deep breathing exercises, meditation, and guided imagery, serve as powerful tools for reducing stress and promoting relaxation. Regular practice of these techniques not only fosters a sense of calm but also enhances resilience in coping with the challenges of recovery. Additionally, engaging in enjoyable activities, such as listening to music, reading, or spending time in nature, can provide much-needed distractions and emotional support. Prioritize self-care activities that promote mental and emotional well-being, recognizing their profound impact on the recovery journey.

Rest and Recovery Practices:

Rest is essential for allowing the body to recuperate and heal effectively following stomach surgery. Adequate sleep plays a fundamental role in the recovery process, facilitating tissue repair, hormone regulation, and immune function.

Establishing a consistent sleep schedule and creating a conducive sleep environment, such as minimizing noise and light disturbances, can promote restorative sleep. Moreover, incorporating periods of rest throughout the day, especially during the initial phases of recovery when fatigue may be pronounced, is crucial for conserving energy and facilitating healing. Balance rest with light activity to prevent prolonged periods of inactivity, which can lead to muscle weakness and delayed recovery. Additionally, prioritize relaxation techniques, such as progressive muscle relaxation or aromatherapy, to enhance relaxation and alleviate tension. Recognize the importance of listening to your body's cues and adjusting activity levels accordingly to optimize the recovery process.

adopting lifestyle tips for recovery post-stomach surgery is integral to achieving optimal healing outcomes and long-term wellness.

Incorporating gentle exercise suggestions, stress management techniques, and rest and recovery practices not only accelerates the healing process but also promotes physical, mental, and emotional well-being. By prioritizing self-care and implementing these strategies, individuals can navigate the recovery journey with greater resilience, ensuring a smoother transition to post-surgery life.

CONCLUSION

the journey of stomach surgery recovery demands meticulous attention to nutrition, meal planning, and overall well-being. Through the comprehensive guidance provided in the "Wholesome Healing Cookbook for Optimal Surgery Recovery," individuals embarking on this path can find solace and support in every stage of their healing process.

From the very outset, the importance of preparation is underscored, with insights into stocking the kitchen, understanding essential tools, and mastering meal planning strategies.

As readers progress through the chapters, they are equipped with invaluable nutritional knowledge tailored specifically to post-surgery needs, including a deep dive into macronutrients, micronutrients, and portion control.

The heart of the cookbook lies in its array of healing recipes, meticulously crafted to provide nourishment, comfort, and satisfaction. From soothing soups and broths to gentle and digestible meals, each dish is thoughtfully designed to support recovery while tantalizing the taste buds.

Moreover, the flexibility of the cookbook shines through in its customization options, catering to diverse dietary preferences and restrictions, ensuring that no individual is left behind on their journey to optimal health.

As readers navigate through the chapters addressing symptom management, reintegration of solid foods, and lifestyle tips for recovery, they are empowered with practical strategies to navigate the challenges inherent in the healing process.

In essence, the "Wholesome Healing Cookbook for Optimal Surgery Recovery" transcends its role as a mere collection of recipes, emerging as a steadfast companion and guide on the road to recovery.

With its wealth of knowledge, delicious recipes, and holistic approach to healing, it stands as an indispensable resource for anyone seeking swift rehabilitation and nourishment post-surgery.

www.ingramcontent.com/pod-product-compliance
Lightning Source LLC
Chambersburg PA
CBHW070814290526
45795CB00002B/718